FOURTH EDITION

Reading Research

A User-Friendly Guide for Nurses and Other Health Professionals

Barbara Davies, RN, PhD
Associate Professor
School of Nursing
Faculty of Health Sciences
University of Ottawa

Jo Logan, RN, PhD
Adjunct Professor
School of Nursing
Faculty of Health Sciences
University of Ottawa

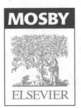

MOSBY
ELSEVIER

Library and Archives Canada Cataloguing in Publication

Davies, Barbara
    Reading research: a user-friendly guide for nurses and other health professionals / Barbara Davies, Jo Logan. — 4th ed.

ISBN-13: 978-0-7796-9990-2   ISBN-10: 0-7796-9990-4

1. Nursing—Research—Evaluation.   2. Medicine—Research—Evaluation.
3. Nursing literature—Evaluation.   4. Medical literature—Evaluation.
I. Logan, Jo   II. Title.

R852.D38 2007   610.73072   C2007-900829-1

Vice-President and Publisher: John Horne
Publisher – Education: Ann Millar
Managing Developmental Editor: Martina van de Velde
Managing Production Editor: Lise Dupont
Copy Editor: Kelly Davis
Cover, Interior Design: Sonya V. Thursby, Opus House Inc.
Typesetting and Assembly: Jansom
Printing and Binding: Printcrafters Inc.

Elsevier Canada
905 King Street West, 4th Floor, Toronto, ON, Canada M6K 3G9
Phone: 1-866-276-5533
Fax: 1-866-359-9534

Printed in Canada

2 3 4 5   12 11 10 09 08

Contents

About the Authors

BARBARA DAVIES, RN, PhD, is an Associate Professor of the University of Ottawa, School of Nursing, and teaches in both the undergraduate and graduate programs. She is the Co-Director of the Nursing Best Practice Research Unit, a collaborative endeavour between the University of Ottawa and the Registered Nurses' Association of Ontario. She received a Premier's Research Excellence Award from the Ministry of Enterprise, Opportunity and Innovation of Ontario, Canada (2004–2009). Her research program aims to increase the transfer and uptake of evidence into practice for front-line healthcare workers, decision makers, and consumers. She is actively involved in the development, implementation, and evaluation of best practice guidelines in nursing and health care.

JO LOGAN, RN, PhD, is an Adjunct Professor of the University of Ottawa, School of Nursing, where she taught in the undergraduate and graduate programs. She is an affiliate member of the Ottawa Health Research Institute and is a member of KT ICEBERG, a research group to enhance capacity for knowledge transfer in health care. Her research interests include evidence-based practice and supportive care, including decision support technology. She is co-developer of the Ottawa Model of Research Use. She has presented numerous workshops on professional practice and research use and was a Director of Nursing Research, Education, and Quality Improvement at the Ottawa Civic Hospital.

Preface

With this new edition, we have continued to keep things simple and user-friendly. As before, this primary guide is about reading research. The intent is to help nurses and other health professionals find and begin to understand health research literature. Complex research concepts are explained in a simpler language. Examples are provided for the beginner and for those seeking a refresher on the meaning of key terms and how to think critically and creatively about research.

In the four years since the previous edition of this book, it has become much easier to access research articles using the Internet. We have expanded the information about searching for research articles with tips for the selection of key search terms. The methods section has been divided into qualitative and quantitative sections, part 1 and part 2, for improved clarity. We have also added a new glossary to help readers quickly find terms.

Throughout the new edition, you will still find **Tips** and **Alerts** that give practical advice to consider when reading research. We do not include examples of research articles in this book because they would soon be out of date and may not be pertinent to all health professions.

One way to use this guide is to select a research article and follow the Reader's Companion Worksheets on pages 39 and 45 as you read the article. If you are a workshop leader, consider selecting articles on hot priority topics that may be of interest to your group for reading in advance of your workshop.

We hope that you will be able to use this guide to understand intriguing research reports that are useful to your studies or work, whether it be in clinical practice, administration, or education. By reading research, using it when appropriate to inform client care, and sharing the new ideas with your colleagues, the health care you provide will improve. This process can create a feeling of excitement and pride. Your new knowledge will provide you with the power to make a difference.

BARBARA DAVIES
JO LOGAN

Acknowledgements

The authors are grateful to the following individuals for their constructive advice on this fourth edition:

Janet Bryanton, RN, BN, MN, PhD Candidate, Assistant Professor, School of Nursing, University of Prince Edward Island, Charlottetown, Prince Edward Island

Zoe Dams, RN, BSN, MSN, Nurse Educator, School of Nursing, Malaspina University College, Nanaimo, British Columbia

Dr. Ian Graham, Vice-President Knowledge Transfer, CIHR, Associate Professor, School of Nursing, University of Ottawa & Associate Director, Clinical Epidemiology Program, Ottawa Health Research Institute, Ottawa, Ontario

Virginia E. Hayes, RN, PhD, Professor, School of Nursing, University of Victoria (Lower Mainland Campus), Vancouver, British Columbia

Debora L. Hogan, RN, BScN, BAPsych, MScN, Research Coordinator, Ottawa Health Research Institute, University of Ottawa Centre for Transfusion Research, Ottawa, Ontario

Jean Jackson, RN, BScN, BPsych, MEd, Coordinator PN Program, Durham College, Oshawa, Ontario

June Kaminski, RN, BSN, MSN, PhD Candidate, Nurse Educator, Faculty of Nursing, Kwantlen University College, Surrey, British Columbia

Nicole Letourneau, RN, PhD, Associate Professor, Faculty of Nursing, University of New Brunswick & Research Fellow, Canadian Research Institute for Social Policy, Fredericton, New Brunswick

Madonna Manuel, RN, BN, NP, MN, Nurse Educator, Western Regional School of Nursing, Corner Brook, Newfoundland

Judy Rashotte, RN, PhD(C), CNCCP(C), Director, Nursing Research & Knowledge Transfer Consultant, Children's Hospital of Eastern Ontario, Ottawa, Ontario

Elizabeth Richard, BScN, MN, RN, Chair, Department of Nursing Education, Grande Prairie Regional College, Grande Prairie, Alberta

Joan E. Tranmer, RN, PhD, Assistant Professor, School of Nursing, Queen's University & Director, Nursing Research Unit, Kingston General Hospital, Kingston, Ontario

1 Introduction

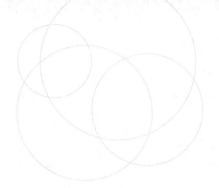

Using research results to inform practice is an essential skill. Government organizations and the public expect that healthcare practitioners, administrators, and policymakers will use research results for the planning and delivery of care. Research has the potential to improve the quality of health care and create "best practices" for patient safety. For example, recent research on factors to consider for the prevention of falls in the elderly has reported the benefits of conducting a risk assessment and providing strength training. By keeping abreast of research results, healthcare practitioners and managers can help senior citizens to avoid falls and potentially serious consequences. Of course, individual clinician judgement and client preferences remain critical to making decisions about the provision of health care.

> tip   Research results are produced constantly, so clinical practice needs to change accordingly.

WHY READ RESEARCH ARTICLES?

- Find solutions to clinical problems
- Find strategies to improve outcomes
- Learn client perspectives
- Acquire new ideas about upcoming technologies
- Find cost-effective practices
- Satisfy professional and personal interests

There are several other reasons to read research articles besides impressing your colleagues, teachers, and managers with your new knowledge. The main reason to read research articles is to have up-to-date, scientifically sound information in order to provide the best client care. Research provides the latest information, and you do not want your knowledge base to be incomplete or obsolete. For example, you may read about an innovative study of an intervention to better manage children's pain or to prevent postpartum depression. If you think that the article has some merit, you may find yourself discussing the findings with your colleagues. As your ability to read research results and to use them appropriately increases, you will be rewarded with the confidence you gain from knowing that you are providing state-of-the-art care.

Another reason to read research is that clients are increasingly aware of research findings, and you need to be on top of the latest evidence in order to assist them in understanding what they've read. There is a growing body of research that comes from grassroots initiatives on topics such as environmental health. Consumer perspectives in healthcare planning and program evaluation are needed, and research articles contain relevant data for planning the most cost-effective and "caring" health services.

In today's competitive and multidisciplinary healthcare system, there is an increased demand for evidence of each profession's contribution to health care and patient outcomes. Reading research will assist you in gaining knowledge that enhances your own professional development. In addition, professional standards require **evidence-based practice** (based on research and other systematic information) whenever possible. And finally, it's fun and inspiring to read a great piece of research.

SOME FRIENDLY ADVICE ABOUT READING RESEARCH ARTICLES

Start reading! It is true that research articles are not usually light reading. The process can be slow and tedious, sometimes even dreary. The language that researchers use, especially in the statistical sections, may seem alien to you. Many people think that they will not understand research reports, so they avoid reading them.

tip	A good dose of skepticism helps when you are reading research articles.

Do not give up on reading research even before you begin, and try not to give up after the first article. It will get easier if you continue reading slowly and thoroughly. It takes practice to read and understand research reports. Like all professional skills, reading research articles is one you can acquire and improve with time. Do not let the report overwhelm you, not even the statistical sections. Just read and understand what you can, then consult with your colleagues and research facilitators about anything that is not clear. They may be able to help you, though there will be times when everyone agrees that a report is confusing. It is important to keep in mind that if you cannot understand some parts of a publication, it may be due to poor writing—not poor reading.

alert! All studies are not created equal.

The quality of the study is critical. As with anything, things can be done right or not so right. The research methods used are especially important— the greater the risk of harm to the participants, the stronger the methods must be.

alert! It is critical that patient safety never be compromised when considering a change in practice.

CHECK OUT THE READER'S COMPANION WORKSHEETS

This book includes two worksheets on pages 39 and 45 for reading research articles. These provide straightforward directions for reading and evaluating quantitative and qualitative research articles. The worksheets are also posted on the book's accompanying Web site for easy downloading. We suggest that you read Chapter 2 and your research article first, then use the appropriate worksheet to help you evaluate the study.

2 Easy Steps for Reading Research

The following is a basic outline of how a research article is organized and includes a description of the important elements that are usually present within the article. It is hoped that you will use this as a map to guide you through the research maze. Articles generally contain these headings: abstract, introduction, methods, results or findings, and discussion. Do not be surprised if the headings in the article you are reading are slightly different, though; practically every journal has its own editorial format.

For many sections, we have suggested questions to ask yourself to make the process of reading and evaluating a research article easier. The section on research methods includes the two main research approaches: qualitative and quantitative.

 tip In the beginning, you might find it useful to read the abstract, introduction, and discussion in order to understand the major aspects of the research project.

TITLE

Presents the topic of the study

1. Does the topic look appealing?
2. Is the topic related to your interests or practice?

Don't be daunted by the titles of research reports, which may seem long and complex. Scan the title for something of interest to you. Titles may include the nature of the study as well as the client population, methods, interventions, or theory tested.

ABSTRACT

Briefly describes what the researchers did and concluded

1. Would the results be useful in your practice?
2. Are you interested in learning more about the study?

Usually, the answers to these questions can be found quickly in the abstract at the beginning of most research articles. If, after looking at this summary, you decide the topic is interesting or similar to the issues you face in your setting, continue to read the rest of the article to review it more closely and decide if the information is of value to you.

INTRODUCTION

Outlines the background of the problem or issue being examined, summarizes the existing literature on the subject, and states the research question, objectives, and possibly the hypotheses

1. What is the problem being presented?
2. What is the research purpose or question?
3. What are the central concepts or variables (e.g., pain, self-esteem)?
4. Is there an underlying theory or conceptual framework?
5. Are most of the references recent, that is, less than 5 years old?
6. Are other articles written by experts cited as sources?

Research articles begin with a description of the problem and the rationale for the study. If you do not understand what the study is about, don't give up yet! It may become clearer as you continue to read. Even if the research question is not clearly stated, the study itself may be of value, so keep reading. This introductory section presents the central **concepts** or the aspects of interest that were selected by the investigator. Concepts can be broadly defined or precisely defined as **variables** so that the characteristics can be measured. The researcher must explain how the variables were measured. Sometimes information about variables is included in the methods section in the description about data collection. In some studies, researchers test a **hypothesis**. The hypothesis states the predicted relationship between two or more variables related to the treatment.

The article should contain a literature review describing what is known about the topic and the gaps in knowledge. Studies should build on existing theory or develop new theory. In some situations, theoretical groundwork may not exist yet. As for the references, there may be several older and important classic ones listed, but most should be recent. After reading a few studies on the subject, you will begin to recognize the names of the experts in that field as these will be the most frequently cited authors. Due to publication length restrictions, the literature review section may be abbreviated.

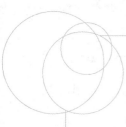

Human Rights Protection

All research requires ethical review and approval. Look for ethical issues while you are reading the report. You may find only one or two sentences about ethical considerations. Sometimes due to editorial restrictions, these details may be excluded entirely. However, it is important to keep ethics in mind, especially if you think you might use the study results in your practice.

Ask yourself the following:
- Is the process of obtaining informed consent mentioned?
- Do you think the participants are vulnerable (e.g., not physically/mentally competent to participate appropriately in the study)?
- Could the intervention have been harmful or potentially harmful to the participants?
- Can you think of any ethical principles that are ignored (e.g., truthfulness, confidentiality)?

METHODS

Describes the techniques used to conduct the study, including design, sample, setting, and data collection and analysis; that is, the "how"

> tip Research articles vary considerably in the order in which the following study techniques are described . . . so be prepared to dig for the information.

Design

The overall plan for answering the research question

1. What is the research approach? Are quantitative, qualitative, or a combination of methods used in the study?
2. What is the research design or plan to answer the research question?

> tip Some articles fail to note what design was used but still may provide valuable information, so keep reading.

Simply defined, quantitative designs involve analyzing numbers in order to answer the research question. Qualitative designs analyze words, observations, or pictures and describe their meanings in order to answer the research question. There are some important differences between qualitative and quantitative designs: underlying beliefs about the nature of reality differ, as do the data analysis methods and the standards for choosing a **sample** and sample size. Designing research is a specialty in itself, and it is virtually impossible to have a perfect design in clinical practice research. When no design is stated, the article should provide the research purpose and methods, so it is still possible to understand how the study was conducted. Researchers may work within a particular ideological framework, such as feminism or critical theory. For example, **feminist research** may use one of any number of designs to examine how gender influences women's and men's lives. **Critical theory** uses philosophical reflection to critique dominant ideas for social and cultural change.

> tip   Look up unfamiliar terms in a glossary or on the Internet.

Part 1: Qualitative Design Methods

Results from qualitative methods can alter our preconceptions about illness experiences or clients' feelings. They can help us understand meanings within other cultures or among religions and genders. For example, studies have been done on grief, immigrant experiences with health care, and the suffering caused by HIV/AIDS. **Qualitative research** tries to make sense of everyday life as it unfolds, without manipulating it.

Qualitative designs focus on research questions that investigate the meanings of a social or human issue within a particular context in order to build a complex holistic picture. These designs are often used when little is known about a topic. They use **inductive analysis** (i.e., working from specific data to broader, more abstract conclusions) and flexible strategies to study perceptions and experiences of people in order to gain in-depth understanding.

Phenomenology research focuses on the meaning of people's experiences concerning some phenomenon. Researchers seek the essence of the phenomenon under study. Phenomenology is based on a philosophy that accepts that an individual's *perception* of an experience is what matters. Perceptions define the reality of the lived experience for a person. During

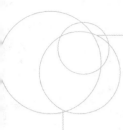

> ## Common Qualitative Designs
>
> - Phenomenology research (philosophy/psychology)—describes a lived (everyday) experience
> - Grounded theory (sociology)—develops theory that is based (grounded) on the data
> - Ethnography research (anthropology)—examines cultures or subcultures
> - Participatory action research (critical social theory/conflict theory)—aims to empower and solve problems*
> - Case study (urban studies, political science)—understands social phenomena within specific real-life contexts*
> - Historical research (history)—discovers facts and relationships of past events*
>
> *These research designs may be used with either qualitative or quantitative design methods.

data collection, investigators and participants may engage in an in-depth conversation. Topics best suited to this approach are fundamental human life experiences, such as the meaning of a parent's death or women's experiences with birthing.

Grounded theory aims to account for patterns of behaviour relevant to the study participants. Data are collected and analyzed concurrently by **constant comparison** of new data to the information already collected and to the developing theory. As the theory is being developed, a core category or concept emerges. The category properties and the relationships among concepts are verified by theoretical sampling (i.e., flexibly selecting sources of data that can add to understanding the pattern).

Ethnography research seeks to understand the world view of participants. This usually involves lengthy observational fieldwork within the cultural setting of interest. Data are interpreted based on the participants' meanings of actions and events. Field notes are made during the observation and a **thick description**, or very detailed account, of cultural behaviours and practices is written. An intensive care unit would be an intriguing example of a subculture that could be studied using this design.

Participatory action research is a type of action research that focuses on engagement between researchers and individuals of communities or groups to work together to generate both new knowledge and change in order to solve an identified problem. In participatory action research, empowerment or freedom from oppressive influence that has become part of the status quo is a goal. Researchers and those who identify a problem and perceive a need for change collaborate equally in the research process—from the study's conception to its conclusion. This approach provides a way to study the problem systematically and solve it by taking action that is relevant to the participants and the people with the problem. An example of a study topic might be spousal battering.

A **case study** is an in-depth study of a "case." The case may be a single person or a group. It could also be an institution, such as a hospital, or a community. The case is usually an incident that is "bounded," or limited, rather than an entity that lacks specificity. For example, the closure of a clinical unit could be the case for a study. The case may be complex or simple, but it is an integrated system. The case is examined in depth by detailing its context and ordinary activities, and the study tries to understand issues related to the history, development, or circumstances of the case.

Historical research looks for patterns and trends among past events and their relevancy to the present. There are several forms of historical research, for example, biographical or social histories. Historians often use written or visual material for data but may also use physical objects from the past. Naturally, the authenticity of the data source is of critical importance to the study. Past nursing practices can be examined through historical methods. For instance, experiences faced by the first public health nurses or perspectives about the first blood transfusions are fascinating and informative.

You will sometimes see general terms used to describe a qualitative study, such as *descriptive qualitative*, rather than one of the common designs. You will see also other qualitative designs not discussed in this primer, for example, *narrative inquiry*, which uses individuals' stories to get at meaning. Check out some of the textbooks in the bibliography for more information on this and other designs that you come across.

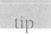
tip

You may want to start your research reading adventures with qualitative studies as the quotations in the results section make research come alive and are easier to understand than some statistical techniques used in quantitative studies.

Rigour in Qualitative Studies

In studies, the issue of rigour (quality) is very important. Rigour refers to the steps taken to ensure that we can be confident that the study results are trustworthy. For a qualitative study, steps are taken to check, question, and theorize. Of course, the significance of the study topic and its relevance to practice and new knowledge are very important. The sample, data collection, and analysis methods should fit the research question and design. The procedures to ensure rigour or **trustworthiness** should be described. Steps should be taken to strengthen study rigour at the time of data collection (e.g., tape-recording interviews). The sample and setting should be described in detail (thick description). Quotations or examples from the data should be provided for you to judge the quality of the investigator's interpretation. New methods for evaluating qualitative studies are emerging, so you will see different steps described, and some will be specific to the design used. For example, **bracketing** is a technique used in phenomenology to identify the researcher's preconceptions about the topic in order to suspend them and set his or her views of the subject aside.

Sample and Setting

Describes the participants in the study and where the study took place

1. What are the characteristics of the participants (e.g., age, gender, experience)?
2. What are the procedures for choosing participants (i.e., how are they selected)?
3. What is the basis for the sample size used?
4. What is the setting where the data were collected (e.g., busy hospital unit, home setting, community)?
5. Does the setting sound similar to one you have experience with?

Qualitative samples are purposely chosen (purposive) for their ability to provide the best information on the study topic. Another sampling technique you will see is "snowball" sampling, which involves asking the first person selected to suggest others. Often, the final size of the sample is determined during data collection, when no new information is being obtained (called data saturation or informational redundancy). The number of participants may be small since there is no need for statistical analysis of numbers; large samples (e.g., a community) are not required but may be used. A case study design may use only one participant or a single organization.

A qualitative study is usually carried out in a natural setting, often called the field (e.g., a patient unit or a community centre). Researchers may spend considerable time gaining access to a setting and do what they can to make the participants feel comfortable about the study and the data collection process. Researchers may be engaged in fieldwork for an extended period of time.

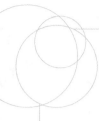

Aspects of Trustworthiness and Qualitative Procedures for Achieving It

- Credibility—What is the truth/reality of the findings? Do they reflect the experiences and perceptions of others? Some techniques used are prolonged field engagement, peer debriefing (with experts), and checking with participants (**member check**). **Triangulation** is the use of several different strategies (i.e., multiple sources of data) to increase rigour.
- Confirmability—Is there *neutrality*, or the absence of bias? Techniques include investigators reviewing their own attitudes or preconceptions about the study topic so they do not impose them on the participants or the data. Keeping a reflective journal and spelling out assumptions helps researchers do this. Recording research process details (**audit trail**) also helps.
- Dependability—Would the data patterns be *consistent*, or stable, over time and for similar conditions? The investigators set up an audit trail of what they did and their results. External persons may be asked to audit the process and findings of the study.
- Transferability—Are the findings *applicable*, important, or useful to a similar group or practice setting? Do the results "ring true" for others? Transferability can be assessed by reviewing examples of the data gathered, often in the form of quotations by participants or detailed thick descriptions.

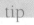 tip
There should be a thorough description of the sample and setting.

Data Collection

Describes the method for gathering the study information

1. What data are collected (e.g., characteristics of participants, photographs, personal experiences, narratives)?
2. How are the data collected (e.g., interview, focus group, observation)?

Qualitative data may be collected from a single source or from multiple sources to help validate the information (triangulation). Qualitative research requires considerable involvement by the researcher, who is the "instrument" of both data collection and analysis. Researchers may collect data by unstructured or semi-structured interviews, **focus groups** (groups of people interviewed together), and observation of the phenomenon of interest and making field notes. Documents can be used as data, for example, letters, diaries, agency policies, or newspaper stories.

Data Analysis and Results

Presents the procedures used to analyze the data and the results or findings

1. What methods of data analysis are used?
2. What are the main research results?
3. Is there a thorough description of the results?

Qualitative data analysis involves working inductively to code the information. The participants' words or metaphors are important starting points. The codes are grouped into broader categories. The categories or conceptual relationships are used to describe or explain the phenomena of interest. You will read studies in which data categories were used to form themes or to generate theory. Figures or diagrams are often used to illustrate ideas. Usually, numbers are used minimally, such as to describe the number of participants (sample) in the study. In qualitative research articles, you may see the findings or results section combined with the discussion section.

tip	Check out the International Institute for Qualitative Methodology: http://www.uofaweb.ualberta.ca/iiqm.

Part 2: Quantitative Design Methods

Quantitative designs in healthcare research use mathematical techniques in order to "quantify" and describe, compare, or predict various aspects related to health, disease, or healthcare services. The aspects or topics that are studied quantitatively are extensive and can include, for example, objects, ideas, blood cells, psychological factors, group behaviours, devices, organizations, or events.

A **deductive approach** is used, which means that researchers use previously known facts or information to construct the methodology. If there has been little previous research about the topic, then foundational descriptive work is usually required, such as a survey. If there has been a considerable amount of previous research, then it is possible to design studies on the predictors of a topic using experimental designs or sophisticated statistical methods.

Predictive **quantitative research** studies have produced important results about phenomena such as low birth weight, middle-age depression, and serious bicycle-related injuries.

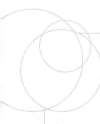

Common Quantitative Designs

Experimental
- Randomized controlled trial (RCT)

Quasi-Experimental
- Pretest–post-test control group (no randomization)

Non-Experimental
- Survey
- Correlational
- Case control
- Cohort study

Experimental Designs

Experiments in healthcare settings are called **randomized controlled trials** (**RCTs**). An individual client or care provider may be the unit of randomization; however, it is becoming more common to randomize groups (e.g., teams, units, institutions), referred to as a *cluster randomized trial*. The experimental group receives special treatment or intervention, such as a teaching program. The researchers are trying to test a hypothesis. The hypothesis states the predicted relationship between two or more variables related to the treatment (e.g., cardiac clients who receive a teaching program about their medications and symptom control will be more confident about their self-care management).

Experimental designs have three essential characteristics:

1. **Randomization** (random assignment of participants to groups)
2. A control group for comparison with the experimental group
3. Manipulation of a special treatment (e.g., early discharge, teaching program)

Quasi-experimental, or in other words "almost experimental," designs lack one or more of the above three characteristics. An example is a **pretest–post-test design**, which does not include randomization of participants. Sometimes in healthcare research it is difficult to design an experiment due to ethical reasons. For example, you would not randomly assign a person to smoke or not smoke.

Non-Experimental Designs

Surveys are used to obtain information from a group or population about a topic of interest. The goal may be to learn how frequently a behaviour is exhibited or to describe and compare attitudes. For example, what are the attitudes of nurses, midwives, and obstetricians about collaborative multidisciplinary maternity care? Please note that using a structured questionnaire with a few open-ended items for the participants to state their views or opinions is not "qualitative" research. While the researcher will use a simplified content coding process similar to methods used in qualitative research, the overall spirit of the study is an attempt to quantify, and thus it is considered a quantitative and not a qualitative study.

Correlational designs focus on describing relationships between factors. Watch for the interpretation of the results in these studies because the researcher is studying factors that already exist, and differences found in the results may be due to self-selection or pre-existing situations. Correlation does not imply causation. Take the example of exercise and weight loss. Factors such as dietary intake, medical history, and physiological parameters need to be considered. Correlational studies are helpful but require detective work by the reader to think about potential alternative explanations.

Case control studies involve matching similar types of clients who receive the treatment (i.e., cases) with clients who do not receive the treatment (i.e., controls). For example, high-risk pregnant women receiving home care (cases) are matched with high-risk pregnant women receiving the usual hospital care (controls). Research is conducted to compare the satisfaction of the women and their families.

A **cohort study** compares two or more different groups over time. An example would be a study to examine the risk of colorectal cancer in people who eat a low-fat, high-fibre diet compared with people who eat a regular diet.

Rigour in Quantitative Studies

As discussed previously, rigour refers to steps taken to ensure that we can be confident that the study results are close to the truth and are not influenced or biased by other factors. Try to think of factors within the particular study (**internal validity**) other than the treatments that might have biased the outcomes. In addition, try to think of factors that occurred during the study that make it difficult to apply the study findings (**external validity**) to other settings, including your own.

  If you think that substantial bias exists, then care must be taken when interpreting or using the research findings.

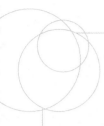

Quantitative Variables

There are three basic types of variables:

1. **Outcome variable** (dependent): the characteristic being measured to find the results (e.g., number of cigarettes smoked, infection rate, level of anxiety)
2. **Experimental variable** (independent): the intervention or treatment being manipulated (e.g., individual vs. group counselling strategies, sterile vs. clean techniques)
3. Other variables (confounding variables, **extraneous variables**): other factors that may influence the results of the study (e.g., age, gender, amount smoked, previous attempts to quit, presence of the researcher, type of hospital, staff available on the unit)

The researcher tries to identify potential confounding variables before beginning the study in order to limit their influence on study outcomes. The potential influence of confounding variables on the results may be controlled either through the research design, statistical techniques, or both. As a clinical practitioner, you are in an ideal position to identify other confounding variables that might have been overlooked by the researcher and may have influenced the study results (e.g., spouse is a heavy smoker).

Sample

Describes the participants in the study

1. What are the characteristics of the group being studied (e.g., age, gender)?
2. What are the conditions for choosing the participants (i.e., who is included/excluded)?
3. Does the study group have characteristics similar to those of clients in your practice (e.g., age, gender, diagnosis, cultural background)?
4. Are there any aspects of the selection of study participants that might have influenced the study outcomes (e.g., geographical location, socio-economic status)?
5. What is the basis for the sample size used?

Sample size is an important consideration. Note the sample size used. Small samples can influence the interpretation of results. Whether 50% of participants equals 10 people out of 20 or 200 out of 400 may make a difference, depending on what is being studied.

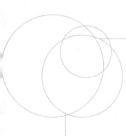

Sources of Bias

Sources of bias are factors that distort study results.

- **Selection bias:** Influences affecting how participants were assigned to study groups (e.g., healthier participants receive the new drug treatment, while less healthy participants receive the usual care)
- **Participation bias:** Influences affecting who participated during the study (e.g., high refusal rate, non-participation of a particular group of people, dropout or death rate)
- **Measurement bias:** Influences affecting how the data were collected (e.g., weight on a scale that is always 2 kg too high, inaccurate blood pressure cuff, non-valid questionnaire)
- **Performance bias** (contamination, co-intervention): Influences affecting the study (e.g., practitioners knowing they were part of the study, participants' awareness of treatments/placebo, additional care to one or both groups that was not intended)

Beware of studies claiming that there is no benefit from one treatment program compared with another treatment program without information about the predetermination of sample size or a description of sample size requirements.

Calculations to determine whether the sample size is sufficient to detect a clinically meaningful difference should be reported in the article. *Power* is the ability of a study to detect meaningful differences. You will see that power is typically set at 0.80.

Sample size estimates are usually calculated on one or two primary outcomes. It is important to know the frequency of the primary outcome in the population under study. Rare outcomes require larger size samples. Carefully think about the primary outcome. Is this a key factor of importance to your work setting?

Data Collection

Describes the method for gathering the study information

1. What data were collected (e.g., characteristics of clients, outcomes, other relevant findings)?
2. What is the setting where the data were collected (e.g., busy hospital unit, home setting, private room, laboratory)?

3. How were the data collected (e.g., questionnaire, interview, auscultation method, observation)?
4. Is there a description of the steps taken to strengthen study rigour (i.e., precision) at the data collection stage (e.g., ensuring reliability and validity of the tools used)?
5. Are there any aspects of the data collection methods that could have influenced the study outcomes (e.g., time of year of data collection, extremely busy unit, biased investigator)?
6. Is there likely to be contamination of treatment across study groups or between clients, families, or healthcare providers?

The **reliability** and **validity** of the study tools are factors associated with rigour. A tool is reliable if it consistently measures what it is supposed to measure, so two people gathering the same data get similar results (**inter-rater reliability**). Another type of reliability is called *test-retest reliability*. In this case, the investigator is trying to determine whether similar results will be obtained if the same tool is used at different times (e.g., one week apart).

A tool is considered valid if it accurately measures what it is intended to measure (e.g., Does it really measure anxiety or is some other feeling being measured?). The number of reliable and valid tools in nursing and allied health is increasing, but there still are not many available. The tool has to be used the same way it was used in other studies in order to keep its validity and reliability. If anything has been changed, it is like trying a new tool. There should be a description of how the tool was tested for reliability and validity—if not, beware.

Two frequently reported characteristics of tools and diagnostic tests are *sensitivity* (how good a test is at detecting who has a condition/disease) and *specificity* (how good a test is at telling who does not have the condition/disease).

Data Analyses and Results

Presents the statistical procedures or the quantitative methods used to analyze the data and the findings

1. What methods of data analysis were used?
2. What are the main research results?

In quantitative studies, the analytical section may be very difficult to interpret without being familiar with statistics or having a statistical background. Read it slowly and more than once. Try to get an idea of what is being said. The following are some key things to consider.

Descriptive Statistics
Express characteristics or summarize data

- The *mean* is the average score.
- The *median* is the score in the middle of a range of scores and is the best indication of a typical score when there are unusually high or low scores.
- The *range* describes the variability and is the difference between the highest and lowest scores.
- *Standard deviation* is another indication of variability and is calculated from the average squared differences (deviations) about the mean.

alert! Extreme or unusual scores have a large influence on the mean, especially if the sample size is small. The median and mean values should be similar. If not, then the median should be used.

Inferential Statistics
Depict inference, relationships, and probabilities
Statistical Significance. Look for the words "statistically significant" in the article. If they are present, it means that the statistical calculation shows a relationship between the variables that is unlikely to be due to just chance. Even though some relationships will occur by chance, researchers want to determine if their study results are most likely due to the experimental intervention rather than chance. Therefore, a **statistically significant** difference will indicate a real difference 95% of the time.

To see if the results are statistically significant, look for "$p \leq 0.05$." This means there is a less than or equal to 5% (0.05) probability (p) that the results found by the researcher are due to chance alone. A very small p-value means that the majority of the observed study results are likely due to the experimental intervention—not to chance.

In tables, statistical significance might be indicated by an asterisk (*) beside some of the numbers. At the bottom of the table, the corresponding note will indicate the p-value. Values of $p \leq 0.05$ and ≤ 0.01 are reported most commonly.

Clinical Relevance. Regardless of statistical significance, it is important to always look at the actual numbers to determine if the results are clinically meaningful. For example, how relevant would it be to your practice if a serious intervention only lowered a patient's temperature by 0.1°C? Results can be statistically significant but not clinically significant, and vice versa.

If results are clinically meaningful but not statistically significant, it could be that the sample size used was too small. If there are a large number of people in the study sample, then statistical significance can be reached more readily. Results with no difference between groups can also be clinically meaningful and may suggest that other options need to be studied.

Confidence Intervals. Is the confidence interval (CI) reported? The **confidence interval** is a range of values within which the true value is expected to be found. The degree of certainty is set by the investigator, usually at 95% and occasionally at 99%. For example, you may read in the newspaper that "A survey reported that 23% of voters agreed to a new scheme. This result is accurate within 4 percentage points 95 times out of 100." What the newspaper report is referring to is the confidence interval, with 23% as the point estimate and ± 4 points as the upper and lower limits. This means that you can be 95% sure that the true value is anywhere from 19% to 27%.

> tip   Reading two or three descriptions of the same term can be helpful to obtain a better grasp of its meaning.

Odds Ratio. Some studies will present information about the odds ratio (OR). An **odds ratio** is the ratio of the odds (likelihood) of an outcome in one group compared with the odds of the outcome in another group. An odds ratio of 1 indicates no difference between groups. If the confidence interval around the odds ratio does not include 1, then the odds ratio is statistically significant.

An example of an odds ratio may help you to understand some of these terms: Women in an experimental group were randomly assigned to receive a treatment, and the odds ratio for a specific adverse event (e.g., increased rate of Caesarean section) was 0.77 with a 95% confidence interval of 0.64 to 0.91. Note that the confidence interval does not include 1; therefore, the treatment group had statistically significant fewer instances of this adverse event.

Correlation. A note about correlation: If two variables are correlated, it does not mean that one caused the other; it means that one variable is related to (associated with) the other variable, either directly or indirectly. For example, height and weight are correlated variables because they are associated, but one does not cause the other. Correlations can be positive or negative, with a range of scores from −1 (negative association) to +1 (positive association). Conventional guidelines used with correlation results (r) often suggest that an r of 0.3 is low while 0.5 is medium and 0.8 is high. But it really depends on the type of variable and the research question. The correlation between two raters observing the same behaviour (inter-rater reliability) should be at least 0.80. Otherwise, you would not know if differences found were due to measurement error or were actual observed behavioural differences.

> alert!   Correlation does not imply causation.

Predictors of Outcomes. **Regression analysis** techniques involve statistical procedures to determine one or more predictors of an outcome (e.g., Is staff retention influenced by factors such as salary, workload, number of night shifts?). Sometimes a theoretical approach is used to select potential factors, and other times an exploratory approach is used. Either a simple or a multiple (many factors at the same time) regression can be done. With a *multiple regression*, the researcher is seeking to know what explains the most variability, called *variance* in the outcome. For example, the presence of leadership, with an r^2 of 0.47, explained a large amount of the variance in whether organizations were able to sustain the implementation of clinical practice guidelines.

Differences in Proportions. **Chi-square test** (χ^2) is a test that compares the actual number with an expected number. It is used when the data are in categories (e.g., male/female, infection/no infection). Look for the differences in proportions over time, such as before and after the initiation of new equipment.

Comparing Mean Scores. A **t-test** is used to analyze the difference between two mean scores, for example, to compare nurses' and respiratory therapists' mean scores of their skill to demonstrate use of inhalation devices.

Analysis of variance (ANOVA) is used to analyze mean score differences between three or more groups. Using the previous example of skills to demonstrate inhaler use, an ANOVA could be done to see whether nurses from emergency, pediatrics, or general medicine have higher scores.

Multivariate analysis of variance (**MANOVA**) is used to compare mean scores of two or more groups on two or more variables at the same time. For example, do confidence scores for managing insulin doses for strenuous exercise and for travel differ between newly diagnosed people with diabetes and those having diabetes for more than two years?

It is beyond the scope of this beginner guide to discuss more statistical tests. However, if you are interested in learning more, we encourage you to check out the textbooks listed on page 37 or statistical and research Web sites and research glossaries. The complexity of analytic techniques is increasing, and newcomers to research and the public cannot be expected to remember or know all of these techniques. In fact, even senior researchers regularly seek expert consultation about statistical methods.

Examples of helpful free sites with information about statistical terms:

* Cochrane Collaboration Glossary:
  http://www.cochrane.org/resources/glossary.htm
* Statnotes: Topics in Multivariate Analysis, by David Garson:
  http://www2.chass.ncsu.edu/garson/pa765/statnote.htm

| tip | Do not hesitate to seek help from others who are knowledgeable about statistics or mathematics. |

Part 3: Combinations of Qualitative and Quantitative Research Methods

It is becoming more and more common for investigators to combine both quantitative and qualitative designs in the same research project (**mixed-method research**). An example of a mixed-method **evaluation research** study can be illustrated with the topic of physical restraints. Research has found that, for most people, physical restraints attached to beds or chairs can actually do more harm than good. A study on the use of physical restraints could quantitatively determine the frequency of physical restraint use by counting the number of patients who are restrained. In addition, the same study could have a second part that seeks to better understand the nurses' feelings about restraint use through qualitative interviews.

One term you may see with mixed-method studies is triangulation. When researchers use multiple sources, methods, or analytic techniques, they may be attempting triangulation for the consideration and validation of results from different dimensions, in order to gain a better understanding of the topic under study.

DISCUSSION

Presents the investigators' explanations of some of their findings and their opinions of what they think their study means for practice and future research

1. Has the study changed or confirmed your thinking on the topic?
2. Do you agree with the opinion of the investigator(s)?
3. Are the results consistent with previous research and practice? If not, are the inconsistencies explained?
4. Does the interpretation make sense theoretically and from a clinical perspective?
5. Can you think of an alternative interpretation?
6. Overall, what are the major strengths and major limitations (weaknesses) of the research?

Both qualitative and quantitative studies conclude with a discussion of the findings and usually provide some implications for practice. The studies may also include implications for the future education of health professionals, theory development, or policy development. The discussion section is usually quite readable and is where you may find good ideas for your own practice, given that your own critique has satisfied you that it was a strong study. If important bias exists, then care must be taken when interpreting or using the research findings. Using research results from quantitative studies in practice may include the application of specific protocols or policies. Qualitative studies may provide new ideas and perspectives to think about and therefore have an effect on practice.

You may feel that you are still struggling with some of the research terms in the article. This is common at first. Reading research reports is a skill and takes ongoing practice. You likely have an opinion about the merit of the study, and your opinion counts. Professionals are consumers of research and are the means through which research gets used in practice.

A FINAL SUGGESTION: THE ACKNOWLEDGEMENTS

Check out the source of funding for any potential conflict of interest that might have had an influence on project design or the interpretation of results. In addition, if you think that conducting research may be of interest to you in your future career, or that graduate education is a possibility for you, pay attention to where researchers obtain funding for their work.

One final aspect to check is the credentials and affiliation of the authors, which may increase your sense of the study's credibility. For major research initiatives, a PhD credential listed for at least one of the authors is expected since a PhD is a research-oriented degree. However, you would also expect to see relevant professional credentials (e.g., OT, PT, RN, MD) indicating clinical expertise within the study team.

3 Finding Interesting Research Results

SEARCHING THE INTERNET

 A search does not need to start inside a library. The Internet can be a quick way to find research articles.

Credibility criteria for Web site information:

- Mission and purpose of the organization stated (to assess your trust of the organization)
- Credentials of authors provided
- Logical and verifiable content
- Systems to maintain accuracy of content
- Content updated regularly
- References included

 Poor-quality Web sites exist. Focus on sites from credible organizations.

Google is a search engine with access to billions of articles and can be helpful, but the results can sometimes be overwhelming and of variable quality. Thus, Google Scholar, which includes only peer-reviewed sources, is recommended when searching for research articles: http://scholar.google.com/.

 Use peer-reviewed sources, which are articles that experts have judged to be acceptable and relevant.

To find out if a journal is peer-reviewed, look for information in the sections entitled "about this journal," "contributor guidelines," or "manuscript submission and review process." You will see words such as "independent review" or "external review," which means that people other than the paid editorial staff are judging the merit and relevance of the research study for publication. You may also see the term "blind peer review," which means that identifying information about the author(s) has been removed before the review process, so the expert reviewer is "blind" to the name of the author(s) and the place/institution where the study was conducted. This helps reviewers to be objective.

The journals listed on page 38 include peer-reviewed articles. Not all current articles are available electronically, and many older ones are not, so sometimes it will be necessary to go to the library or request interlibrary retrieval.

alert!   Not all journals or selected papers are peer-reviewed!

Portals

The Public Health Agency of Canada operates The Canadian Best Practices Portal for Health Promotion and Chronic Disease Prevention. It is free and includes many references and articles. You can even e-mail an expert from this portal for advice on your topic: http://cbpp-pcpe.phac-aspc.gc.ca/index_e.cfm.

The Canadian Nurses Association (CNA) manages a bilingual Web portal (NURSEONE) with information vetted by their review committees. The portal is free for nurses or student nurses who are members of CNA through their provincial associations. The portal includes many databases for searching (e.g., CINAHL, Medline, and **Cochrane Collaboration**, a database of systematic reviews), and you can save your personal search strategies: http://www.nurseone.ca/.

The MDLinx Company offers a free Internet-based resource for medical and other health professionals and patients. Easy, quick access is provided to popular journal articles, professional association resources, and consumer groups. This site has search capabilities and includes links for medicine, pharmacology, and NurseLinx: http://www.nurselinx.com/.

tip   Try to find two to three articles on a similar topic to get a sense of the field.

SEARCHING BIBLIOGRAPHIC DATABASES

The most efficient way to search for research articles is to access databases. The trick to finding relevant articles is to identify the key words or terms used for the search. Use the "Help" feature in each database to obtain the best search results. A librarian can also help you select key terms and describe the logic commands for a good search. If you already have a few articles on the topic, take them to show the librarian the key words used. Keep in mind that it may take several searches using different terms and databases to achieve a thorough review of the literature. Look for the catalogue of databases available electronically.

The following is a list of suggested bibliographic databases:

- CINAHL (nursing and allied health)
- EMBASE (biomedical and pharmaceutical)
- Medline (medicine, life sciences, and biomedical)
- PsychInfo (psychology and related disciplines)
- Cochrane Collaboration (medical and healthcare systematic reviews)

tip   To do a thorough search, ask a librarian for help.

If you are working on a special project, a librarian may be able to suggest resources that you are not familiar with. During the project, the librarian might be willing to be on the lookout for you for new helpful sources.

SEARCH TERMS

Think carefully about potential search terms that are focused and reflect the essence of your project or query. Most databases will have subject headings that are pre-designated (e.g., MeSH, or medical subject headings, a vocabulary established by librarians). You just need to pick a few headings that are the most suitable.

Example: pain management for palliative care of cancer clients in the home

Search of CINAHL: Click on the subject heading to review the dimensions of the term.

- *Pain: e.g., cancer pain, pain management, pain level, symptom severity*

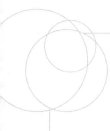

Tips for Managing Your Search (Boolean Logic)
- Insert "AND" to limit your search by combining terms where two or more topics must overlap.
- Insert "OR" to expand your search.
- Insert "NOT" to exclude items.
- Consider applying limits to your search, such as type of article (e.g., research only), language, and publication date.
- To better focus your results, you can search using any text word that can be found in the title or abstract, but watch out for using common terms from the abstract, such as "support."

- *Palliative Care: e.g., oncologic care, terminal care*
- *Home Care: e.g., home health care, home nursing care, home nursing professional*

Look at the number of hits that you get when you enter the terms—this will help you to focus your search. It is not reasonable to have to go through hundreds of papers at your beginner level.

HOW FAR BACK SHOULD I SEARCH?

This is a common question, but not always an easy one to answer. A reasonable answer is five years. However, if substantive research led to recent practice changes (e.g., hormone therapy for menopausal women or Caesarean section for breech presentation), then a search for the previous two or three years might be sufficient. For a very thorough search by someone with lots of time, a ten-year perspective would be helpful. Start your reading with the most recent article.

KEEPING UP TO DATE

One way of keeping current with new ideas in your area of client care is to regularly scan the table of contents of your favourite or pertinent journals and note any articles that seem to be interesting or related to your practice. Many journals will e-mail the table of contents to you free of charge.

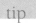 tip   Have the table of contents of your three favourite journals e-mailed to you, to help you keep up to date.

4 Using Research Results

1. Do you think the research findings *should* be implemented into practice?
2. Do you think you *could* implement the recommendations in your practice?

The purpose of reading research is to challenge yourself with new ideas and to continuously improve care by using research findings. **Research utilization** is the application of study findings to practice or policy. There are different ways to use research. You can use it at a conceptual level, in which you reflect on the research findings. For example, you might observe your clients to see if the research findings about establishing and maintaining therapeutic relationships fit with your practice. Another way to use research is at a practical level, in which you actually change your practice and provide care in a different way, for example, by altering the care provided to clients with venous leg ulcers.

A conceptual example for the topic of therapeutic relationship—a clinician's comment:

> I always feel I relate fairly well to my patients. It [the research report] did bring up a few things, and it made me more aware. I just think I'm a little bit more aware of what I do and how I approach people. It's had some effect. I'm sure it just made me think more wisely, I suppose, or more broadly, really.

A practical example for the topic of care of venous leg ulcers—a clinician's comment:

> The patients notice that different things are being done and the wound is now healing. They say, "I feel better. You know, I felt like garbage for the past year and a half. I couldn't walk, and now I'm walking with my grandkid again."

alert! Applying research is always combined with practitioner judgement and client input.

THE QUESTIONS TO ASK

Once you feel somewhat comfortable with the information in the research article, ask yourself the following questions:

1. Is the study potentially helpful to your practice by
   - giving you insights into clients' views of health and illness?
   - providing new ways to assess client/family needs?
   - improving healthcare procedures and interventions?
   - suggesting the need for **quality improvement**?
   - enhancing the quality of work life?
   - providing information for education programs?
   - providing care more quickly or efficiently?
2. Would the application of the results be consistent with current healthcare agency policies, procedures, and standards?
   - Are new policies, procedures, standards, or medical directives needed?
   - Will patient safety be maintained?
3. Would it be reasonable to implement the study findings if
   - the clients or healthcare providers are similar to your setting?
   - the findings would be acceptable to administrators, colleagues, or other disciplines in your organization?
   - the costs are not a hindrance?
4. Is the benefit to clients worth the effort of obtaining the resources necessary to make the change? What are the barriers? If the research findings suggest a new direction for client care that requires a change in policies, procedures, or standards, consider the following:
   - Knowledge/skills and attitudes of "pertinent players"
   - Equipment and staff availability
   - Time and money
5. How strong is the research design in relation to the required change of practice?

All research designs have value, but some research designs are better suited to one purpose than another. With regard to clinical interventions, therapies, and treatments, research designs are ranked hierarchically, with the designs that provide the most predictive evidence as the strongest levels. For example, for the research question "Does the use of an asthma action plan help with control of symptoms?" a randomized controlled trial is the best design to compare treatments. The results of descriptive surveys and qualitative studies are important to provide knowledge about the clients' perspectives or the healthcare environment, but they are not used to compare one intervention with another to see which has the best effect.

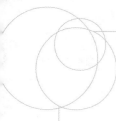

Levels of Evidence*

- Systematic reviews of multiple randomized controlled trials (experiments)
- Single experiments
- Quasi-experimental studies
- Non-experimental research, including qualitative studies
- Quality management databases
- Consensus of respected authorities

*The levels of evidence are listed as a hierarchy, with the strongest evidence for implementing interventions or treatments at the top.

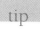 All types of research evidence provide valuable information for understanding the context of health care.

 Levels of evidence and quality ratings of studies vary. Be sure to check the authors' numerical ratings as the scoring is not universal. Not all hierarchies go from top to bottom; sometimes scores/levels are categorized uniquely and may even be reverse-ordered.

THE DECISION TO USE RESEARCH RESULTS

 If you can link your desired change in practice to patient safety and quality improvement, you are likely to get more support from others.

The decision to use research findings in your practice requires that you consider the following:

- If you identify the need for a change in practice that requires new or revised policies, procedures, or standards, or if the change exceeds your responsibilities, then share the information with your teacher, clinical resource person, managers, or other administrators.
- Always keep in mind the effect of changing clinical practice on client safety. Before you put the study results into practice, talk with your

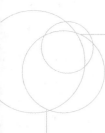

Types of Reviews

- **Integrative review:** A review of the literature that assimilates the results of research studies by comparing and contrasting them in order to describe the state of knowledge. It may include quantitative and qualitative research studies.
- **Systematic review:** A synthesis or combination of quantitative research studies on clearly defined questions that uses explicit methods for finding and appraising research. Usually, the goal is to summarize the effect of an intervention. Commonly, but not always, it uses meta-analytic techniques.
- **Meta-analysis:** A statistical technique to combine the results of several quantitative studies together to determine if overall the intervention had an effect or not.
- **Meta-synthesis:** An integration and summary of the findings of qualitative studies on a given topic.
- **Evidence-based clinical practice guideline:** A review of research on a topic with the purpose of making explicit recommendations for practice.

colleagues, managers, researchers, and other health professionals to see if they agree with the change.

- Practice is seldom changed on the basis of one study. Fortunately, there are increasing numbers of research syntheses available to busy clinicians who wish to practice according to research rather than by tradition or habit.

Authors of integrative review articles are frequently experts in the field, but the articles selected to be in the review and the interpretation of the results are shaded by the writers' views and experiences. If you want to read more, you can find the original papers (primary sources) written by the researchers.

An integrative review article is another person's interpretation of the original research and is often referred to as a secondary source.

CLINICAL PRACTICE GUIDELINES

A really useful synthesis is in the form of a **clinical practice guideline**. Also called best practice guidelines, these documents present recommendations that are based on a rigorous review of many studies by experts on the topic.

You should note that the strength or quality of evidence may vary for each recommendation within a guideline. Remember that the quality of clinical or best practice guidelines should be evaluated before you use the recommendations.

Decision makers in healthcare organizations who strive to ensure high-quality, up-to-date services are establishing systems for the ongoing review and revision of policies and procedures. Increasingly, they are using best practice guidelines to help keep current with research-based recommendations from international, national, and provincial groups. Following is a list of credible guideline Web sites to get you started.

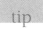 tip | Look for clinical practice guidelines or systematic reviews from a credible journal or organization.

Practice Guideline Web Sites

This list is a starting point. You will find many more Web sites at www.elsevier.ca/ReadingResearch/.

- The Joanna Briggs Institute (Australia):
  http://www.joannabriggs.edu.au/about/home.php
- National Guideline Clearinghouse (United States):
  http://www.guideline.gov
- Centre for Reviews and Dissemination (United Kingdom):
  http://www.york.ac.uk/inst/crd/
- Nursing Best Practice Guidelines, Registered Nurses' Association of Ontario: http://www.rnao.org/bestpractices/

Appraisal of Guidelines for Research and Evaluation

It is beyond the scope of this book to evaluate the quality of evidence summaries, reviews, and guidelines. Evaluating the merits of a combination or group of research studies is more complex than evaluating the merits of a single study. However, if you would like to learn more about these topics, check out the following Web sites:

- AGREE (Appraisal of Guidelines Research and Evaluation): AGREE Instrument (available for free):
  http://www.agreecollaboration.org/instrument/

- Critical Appraisal Skills Program (CASP) and Evidence-Based Practice: Public Health Resource Unit, National Health Service (United Kingdom): http://www.phru.nhs.uk/casp/casp.htm

WANT TO LEARN MORE?

Web site addresses may change, and new sites are continually being developed. For an expanded and up-to-date list, please see this book's accompanying Web site: www.elsevier.ca/ReadingResearch/. You will find many more links there.

Also consider doing some of the following:

- Consult our bibliography and list of peer-reviewed journals.
- Seek research courses at local universities and colleges.
- Ask your agency's education department for speakers, teleconferences, and workshops.
- Contact professional organizations for resources and speakers.
- Invite the author of a research report to speak to your group.
- Form a journal club.
- Become active on agency practice committees.

Glossary

Analysis of variance (ANOVA) p. 20   A statistical test for comparing mean differences in three or more groups by comparing variability between the groups and within each group.

Audit trail p. 11   A process record used in qualitative studies to note the decisions and actions taken.

Bracketing p. 10   A phenomenological research process to identify and suspend any preconceived notions held by the researcher about the study topic.

Case control study p. 14   A design that matches similar types of patients who receive the treatment (i.e., cases) with patients who do not receive the treatment (i.e., controls).

Case study p. 9   A research design that focuses in depth on specific (often small) populations or well-defined events that are bounded by time.

Chi-square test (χ^2) p. 20   A statistical test to assess differences in proportions using data that come from categories.

Clinical practice guideline p. 31   Evidence-based recommendation for care that should be accompanied by practitioner judgement and experience, as well as client preferences.

Cochrane Collaboration p. 25   An international organization for the development and updating of systematic reviews on healthcare effectiveness topics.

Cohort study p. 14   A design involving comparison between participants in two or more different groups (i.e., cohorts) over time.

Concept p. 5   An abstract idea formed by examining specific instances (e.g., grief).

Confidence interval (CI) p. 19   A range of values within which the true value is expected to be found.

Constant comparison p. 8   A grounded theory analysis technique to clarify the developing theory by comparing data as they are collected with previously collected data.

Correlational design p. 14   Examines the statistical interrelationships among variables. Also called correlational research.

Critical theory p. 7   A social theory oriented to the critique of dominant ideas with the intent to create social and cultural change.

Deductive approach p. 12   A quantitative approach applying known facts or theory.

Ethnography research p. 8   Research using a qualitative method, based in anthropology, that focuses on a group's culture to learn its world view.

Evaluation research p. 21   A study to assess how a program, policy, or practice is performing.

Evidence-based practice p. 2   Practice decisions based on reliable and valid research and other systematic information (that should also take into account practitioner experience and judgement and client preferences).

Evidence-based clinical practice guideline p. 31   A review of research on a topic with the purpose of making explicit recommendations for practice.

Experimental variable p. 15   The intervention or treatment being manipulated. Also called independent variable.

External validity p. 14   The extent to which the research results can be generalized or applied to other settings or samples.

Extraneous variable p. 15   A variable that confounds (confuses) the relationship between the independent and the dependent variables.

Feminist research p. 7   Focuses on issues of gender and how they have influenced women and men socially and historically.

Focus group p. 11   A group of individuals interviewed together on a topic common to each of them.

Grounded theory p. 8   Qualitative research that ultimately intends to develop theory from data that are derived (grounded) from real-world examples.

Historical research p. 9   An investigation seeking patterns and trends among past events and their relevancy to the present.

Hypothesis p. 5   A statement that predicts relationships between variables.

Inductive analysis p. 7   The qualitative research process of working from specific observations/data to general conclusions.

Integrative review p. 31   A review of the literature that assimilates the results of research studies by comparing and contrasting them in order to describe the state of knowledge. It may include quantitative and qualitative research studies.

Internal validity p. 14   The extent to which the study design and methodology produce valid accurate results and uncontrolled or extraneous factors are not responsible for the outcomes.

Inter-rater reliability p. 17   The degree to which two people (raters) working independently using the same research tool at the same time get similar results.

Measurement bias p. 16   Influences that affect how the data are collected or coded.

Member check p. 11   A qualitative research validation of credibility obtained by feedback from study participants.

Meta-analysis p. 31   A statistical technique for combining the findings of quantitative studies on a given topic.

Meta-synthesis p. 31   An approach to compare and integrate findings from qualitative studies on a given topic.

Mixed-method research p. 21   Combines both quantitative and qualitative components simultaneously or sequentially in the same research project.

Multivariate analysis of variance (MANOVA) p. 21   A statistical test of the differences between the mean scores of two or more groups on two or more outcome variables considered at the same time.

Odds ratio (OR) p. 19   A ratio of the odds (likelihood) of an outcome in one group compared with the odds of the outcome in another group.

Outcome variable p. 15   The characteristic being measured to find the results. Also called dependent variable.

Participation bias p. 16   Influences affecting the sample that participated in the study.

Participatory action research p. 8   Research in which the researcher and participating group share ownership of a project to investigate a social problem that involves them, with the intent to empower people and solve problems.

Performance bias p. 16   Influences affecting patients or staff participating in a study. Sometimes controlled by using placebos.

Phenomenology research p. 7   Qualitative research, rooted in philosophy and psychology, that describes or interprets the lived experience of people.

Pretest–post-test design p. 13   A design with data collected before (pre) and after (post) the subjects receive an experimental intervention or treatment. Also called before-and-after design.

Qualitative research p. 7   An inductive, in-depth investigation of phenomena in a holistic fashion that uses a flexible research design.

Quality improvement p. 29   A method of evaluating and improving the processes of health care, often using a multidisciplinary approach to problem solving.

Quantitative research p. 12   The investigation of phenomena that uses precise measurement to yield data that are subjected to statistical analysis.

Randomization p. 13   The assignment of participants to study groups based on chance (e.g., using a random numbers table). Each participant has an equal probability of being in each study group.

Randomized controlled trial (RCT) p. 13   An experimental study to test the impact of a new treatment or intervention, with random assignment of participants to a treatment with one or more control or comparison groups. May be carried out on a clinical unit and also called a randomized clinical trial.

Regression analysis p. 20   A statistical test to predict an outcome based on the values of one or more factors.

Reliability p. 17   The extent to which a data collection tool consistently measures the same attribute that it is designed to measure, or the extent to which the results can be replicated.

Research utilization p. 28   The application of study findings to practice or policy.

Sample p. 7   The part of a population that is selected to participate in a study.

Selection bias p. 16   Influences affecting how participants were selected and/or assigned to study groups.

Statistically significant p. 18   The result of a statistical calculation that shows a relationship between the study variables is unlikely to be due to chance alone.

Survey p. 13   Non-experimental research that uses questionnaires or interviews to obtain information such as beliefs, preferences, attitudes, or activities of people.

Systematic review p. 31   A synthesis or integration of research studies.

Thick description p. 8   A detailed account of cultural practices used in ethnography to present results and provide evidence of rigour.

Triangulation p. 11   Using multiple sources (methods, data collection, theories) to help validate information.

Trustworthiness p. 10   Refers to the rigour (quality) associated with the qualitative research process and results.

t-test p. 20   A statistical test used to analyze the difference between two mean scores, for example, to compare nurses' and respiratory therapists' mean scores of their skill to demonstrate use of inhalation devices.

Validity p. 17   The degree to which a data collection tool accurately measures what it is intended to measure.

Variable p. 5   An attribute or characteristic of a person or object that varies (takes on different values).

Bibliography

Here are a few suggestions to get you started if you would like to learn more about research methods.

Burns, N., & Grove, S. K. (2006). *Understanding nursing research: Building an evidence-based practice* (4th ed.). Toronto: W.B. Saunders. ISBN: 1416026401.

LoBiondo-Wood, G., Haber, J., Cameron, C., & Singh, M. (2005). *Nursing research in Canada: Methods, critical appraisal, and utilization*. Toronto: Elsevier. ISBN: 0779699556.

Loiselle, C. G., Profetto-McGrath, J., & Polit, D. (2006). *Canadian essentials of nursing research* (2nd ed.). Philadelphia: Lippincott, Williams & Wilkins. CD-ROM in pocket. ISBN: 0781784166.

Morse, J. M., & Field, P. A. (2003). *Nursing research: The application of qualitative approaches* (2nd ed.). Cheltenham, UK: Stanley Thornes Publishers. ISBN: 0748735011.

Morse, J., & Richards, L. (2002). *Read me first for a user's guide to qualitative methods*. Thousand Oaks, CA: Sage Publications. CD-ROM in pocket. ISBN: 0761918914.

Munhall, P. L. (Ed.). (2007). *Nursing research: A qualitative perspective* (4th ed.). Boston: Jones and Bartlett. ISBN: 0763738646.

Munro, B. H. (2004). *Statistical methods for health care research* (5th ed.). Philadelphia: Lippincott, Williams & Wilkins. ISBN: 0781748402.

Norman, G. R., & Streiner, D. L. (2003). *PDQ pretty darned quick statistics* (3rd ed.). Hamilton, ON: B.C. Decker, Inc. CD-ROM in pocket. ISBN: 1550092073.

Parahoo, K. (2006). *Nursing research: Principles, process and issues* (2nd ed.). New York: Palgrave Macmillan. ISBN: 0333987276.

Polit, D. F., & Beck, C. T. (2003). *Nursing research: principles and methods* (7th ed.). Philadelphia: Lippincott, Williams & Wilkins. ISBN: 0781737338.

Polit, D. F., & Beck, C. T. (2006). *Essentials of nursing research: Methods, appraisal, and utilization* (6th ed.). Philadelphia: Lippincott, Williams & Wilkins. ISBN: 0781749727.

Journals that Publish Peer-Reviewed Research

This list, which is not all-inclusive, is a useful starting point. Some of these journals also have Web sites. For a listing of these, please see this book's accompanying Web site: www.elsevier.ca/ReadingResearch/.

Advances in Nursing Science
American Journal of Critical Care
Applied Nursing Research
Canadian Journal of Nursing Leadership
Canadian Journal of Nursing Research
Canadian Journal of Occupational Therapy
Canadian Journal of Public Health
Canadian Medical Association Journal
Canadian Nurse/L'infirmière canadienne
Cancer Nursing
Clinical Nursing Research
Evidence-Based Nursing
Journal of Advanced Nursing
Journal of Emergency Nursing
Journal of Gerontological Nursing
Journal of Neuroscience Nursing
Journal of Nursing Scholarship
Journal of Obstetric, Gynecologic, and Neonatal Nursing
Nursing Research
Physiotherapy Canada
Qualitative Health Research
Research in Nursing and Health
Respiratory Care
Social Work in Health Care
Western Journal of Nursing Research
Worldviews on Evidence-Based Nursing

Qualitative Research
THE READER'S COMPANION WORKSHEET

Article Title: _____

Author(s): _____

TITLE

Topic of interest	Yes ❑	No ❑	Maybe ❑
Method of interest	Yes ❑	No ❑	Maybe ❑
Population of interest	Yes ❑	No ❑	Maybe ❑

ABSTRACT

Results useful   Yes ❑   No ❑   Maybe ❑

INTRODUCTION

Why is the study being done (i.e., the problem, concern, issue)?

_____

_____

What is the purpose of the study or the question(s) that the investigator is trying to answer (e.g., literature review)?

_____

_____

What are the central concepts (e.g., pain, grief, nursing work)?

_____

_____

Are most of the references recent (less than 5 years old)?   Yes ❑   No ❑
If no, is this a classic/groundbreaking reference or one that has re-emerged in importance (i.e., research relating to tuberculosis)?

_____

Are experts cited?   Yes ❑   No ❑   Not sure ❑

METHODS

Design

What is the research design (e.g., case study, grounded theory, phenomenology, historical research)?

_____

_____

Is the research design appropriate to answer the research question?
Yes ❑   No ❑   Not sure ❑

Sample

What are the characteristics of the participants who were included and excluded from the study (e.g., health status, age, education, gender, ethnicity, occupation, socio-economic status)?

Included: _____

_____

_____

Excluded: _____

_____

_____

Does the selection of the participants fit with the concept being studied?
Yes ❑   No ❑   Not sure ❑

Where were the participants recruited (e.g., self-help group, clinical unit)?

_____

_____

What were the procedures for choosing participants (e.g., purposively selected, snowball technique)?

_____

_____

Human Rights Protection

Was informed consent obtained?   Yes ❑   No ❑
Was the participant reasonably able to take part?   Yes ❑   No ❑
Was the study potentially/actually harmful to participants/others? Yes ❑   No ❑

List any ethical principles ignored (e.g., truthfulness, confidentiality).

_____

_____

Setting

What was the setting in which the data were collected?
Busy unit ❑   Home setting ❑   Private room ❑   Other ❑

Data Collection

What strategy or strategies were used for the data collection?
Focus group ❑   Structured interview ❑   Unstructured interview ❑
Observation ❑   Other ❑ _____

Did the researcher explain his or her role in the data collection process?
Yes ❑   No ❑   Not stated ❑

_____

_____

How were the data recorded (e.g., field notes, tape-recorded, videotaped)?

_____

_____

Was data saturation reached? Yes ❑   No ❑   Not stated ❑   Not applicable ❑

Data Analysis

What methods of data analysis were used (i.e., how were the categories/
themes derived, constant comparison)?

_____

_____

Were the data analyzed inductively?   Yes ❏   No ❏   Not stated ❏

Were strategies used to ensure rigour/trustworthiness?
Yes ❏   No ❏   Not stated ❏
If yes, what were they (e.g., review by others, exemplars provided, audit trail)?

_____

_____

Did the researcher critically examine his or her own role, assumptions, and preconceptions?
Yes ❏   No ❏   Not sure ❏

RESULTS AND DISCUSSION

What are the main findings of the study (i.e., major categories/themes that emerged)?

_____

_____

_____

_____

What information is presented in figures or tables? Are they easy to understand or confusing?

_____

_____

Do you agree with the investigator's interpretation of the results?   Yes ❏   No ❏
If not, why not?

_____

_____

Are the results consistent with past research?   Yes ❏   No ❏   Not applicable ❏
If not, why not?

_____

_____

Does the interpretation make sense theoretically?
Yes ❏   No ❏   Not applicable ❏
If not, why not?

_____

_____

Does the interpretation offer any ideas that you can use?
Yes ❏   No ❏   Not applicable ❏
If not, why not?

_____

_____

OVERALL IMPRESSIONS

Overall, is the article important or significant for the practice of health care?
Yes ❏   No ❏

Do the findings resonate (seem correct and familiar) with you and your practice?
Yes ❏   No ❏
If yes, why?_____

_____

Major limitations of the study (2 or 3):

_____

_____

_____

Major strengths of the study (2 or 3):

_____

_____

_____

Are the results transferable?   Yes ❏   No ❏   Not sure ❏

USING RESEARCH RESULTS

Are the participants similar to those in your setting?
Yes ❏   No ❏   Somewhat ❏

Once you feel somewhat comfortable with the information in the study, ask yourself these questions:

Will information from the study help with the following?

Understanding clients' perspectives: Yes ❑ No ❑ Maybe ❑ Not applicable ❑
Assessment: Yes ❑ No ❑ Maybe ❑ Not applicable ❑
Procedure/protocol: Yes ❑ No ❑ Maybe ❑ Not applicable ❑
Interventions: Yes ❑ No ❑ Maybe ❑ Not applicable ❑
Interpersonal relationships: Yes ❑ No ❑ Maybe ❑ Not applicable ❑
Quality improvement programs: Yes ❑ No ❑ Maybe ❑ Not applicable ❑
Work life/environment: Yes ❑ No ❑ Maybe ❑ Not applicable ❑
Education programs: Yes ❑ No ❑ Maybe ❑ Not applicable ❑
Other:

_____

_____

Are the findings consistent with policies, procedures, and standards?

Require new policy: Yes ❑ No ❑ Not sure ❑
Require new procedure: Yes ❑ No ❑ Not sure ❑
Require new standard: Yes ❑ No ❑ Not sure ❑
Can safety be maintained? Yes ❑ No ❑ Not sure ❑

Do you think the findings are acceptable to the following people?

Clients: Yes ❑ No ❑ Not sure ❑
Administrators: Yes ❑ No ❑ Not sure ❑
Colleagues: Yes ❑ No ❑ Not sure ❑
Other professionals: Yes ❑ No ❑ Not sure ❑

Are the following required for using the results?

Equipment: Yes ❑ No ❑
Staff: Yes ❑ No ❑
Time: Yes ❑ No ❑
Money: Yes ❑ No ❑
Knowledge/skills: Yes ❑ No ❑
Attitude change: Yes ❑ No ❑

Is the benefit worth the effort of obtaining the resources and changing practice?
Yes ❑ No ❑
Why or why not?

_____

_____

Quantitative Research
THE READER'S COMPANION WORKSHEET

Article Title: _____

Author(s): _____

TITLE

Topic of interest   Yes ❑   No ❑   Maybe ❑
Method of interest   Yes ❑   No ❑   Maybe ❑
Population of interest   Yes ❑   No ❑   Maybe ❑

ABSTRACT

Results useful   Yes ❑   No ❑   Maybe ❑

INTRODUCTION

Why is the study being done (i.e., problem, concern, issue)?

_____

_____

What is the purpose of the study or the question(s) that the investigator is trying to answer (e.g., literature review)?

_____

_____

What are the central concepts and variables (e.g., pain level, confidence, exercise activity)?

Concepts under study:

_____

_____

The experimental (independent) variable is defined as:

_____

_____

The outcome (dependent) variable is defined as:

_____

_____

Other variables that the researcher has not thought about that might influence
the results are:

_____

_____

Note that sometimes there are many factors included in descriptive surveys and
not a primary or secondary outcome. If this is the case in the article that you are
reading, provide an overall description.

_____

_____

Are most of the references recent (less than 5 years old)?   Yes ❏   No ❏
If no, is this a classic/groundbreaking reference or one that has re-emerged in
importance (i.e., research relating to tuberculosis)?

_____

Are experts cited?   Yes ❏   No ❏   Not sure ❏

METHODS

Design

What is the research design (e.g., survey, case control, cohort study)?

_____

_____

Sample

What are the characteristics of the participants who were included and excluded
from the study (e.g., health status, age, education, gender, ethnicity, occupation,
geographical residence, socio-economic status)?

Included: _____

_____

_____

Excluded: _____

_____

_____

Are the participants similar to those in your setting?
Yes ❑   No ❑   Somewhat ❑

What are the procedures for choosing participants (e.g., convenience, quota, random selection, volunteers)?

_____

_____

Do you think the methods used to select participants for the study biased the results?
Selection bias   Yes ❑   No ❑
If yes, how?

_____

_____

Were there many refusals, withdrawals, dropouts, or deaths?
Participation bias   Yes ❑   No ❑

_____

_____

Human Rights Protection

Was informed consent obtained?   Yes ❑   No ❑
Was the participant reasonably able to take part?   Yes ❑   No ❑
Was the study potentially/actually harmful to participants/others?   Yes ❑   No ❑

List any ethical principles ignored (e.g., truthfulness, confidentiality).

_____

_____

Setting

What was the environment in which the data were collected?
Home setting ❑   Private room ❑   Laboratory ❑   Other ❑

Experiment (if applicable)

What was the special treatment or intervention?

_____

_____

Did the participants in the study know whether they received the intervention or a placebo?   Yes ❏   No ❏

What methods, if any, were used to "blind" the participants, staff, and data collectors from knowledge about the study that might influence the results?

_____

_____

Was there any contamination or mixing of treatments across the study groups?

_____

_____

Were there any other factors related to the intervention/treatment that might have influenced the outcomes?
Performance bias   Yes ❏   No ❏
If yes, what were they?

_____

_____

Data Collection

What was the data collection method/tool used?
Questionnaire ❏   Interview ❏   Chart review ❏   Procedure ❏
Observation ❏   Other ❏ _____

Were methods used to ensure that data were reliably collected (e.g., differences between raters, differences between times of measurement)?
Yes ❏   No ❏   Not reported ❏
If yes, what were they?

_____

_____

Were methods used to ensure the validity of the collected data (e.g., expert review, comparison with other measures)?
Yes ❏   No ❏   Not reported ❏
If yes, what were they?

_____

_____

Do you think that the measurement methods biased the results?
Measurement bias   Yes ❏   No ❏
If yes, how?

_____

_____

Data Analysis

What statistical methods were used to analyze the data?

_____

_____

RESULTS

Was the response rate satisfactory?   Yes ❏   No ❏   Not sure ❏

What are the main findings of the study?

_____

_____

What information is presented in tables, figures, or graphs? Are these easy to understand or confusing?

_____

_____

Were any of the findings statistically significant?   Yes ❏   No ❏   Not sure ❏
If yes, what were they?

_____

_____

Were there clinically meaningful results/trends?
Yes ❑   No ❑   Not applicable ❑   Not sure ❑
If yes, what were they?

_____

_____

DISCUSSION

Do you agree with the investigator's opinions?   Yes ❑   No ❑   Somewhat ❑
If not, why not?

_____

_____

Are the results consistent with past research?   Yes ❑   No ❑   Not applicable ❑
If not, why not?

_____

_____

Does the interpretation make sense theoretically?   Yes ❑   No ❑   Not sure ❑
If not, why not?

_____

_____

Does the interpretation make sense clinically?   Yes ❑   No ❑   Not sure ❑
If not, why not?

_____

_____

OVERALL IMPRESSIONS

Overall, is the article important or significant for the practice of health care?
Yes ❑   No ❑

Do the findings resonate (seem correct and familiar) with you and your practice?
Yes ❑   No ❑
If yes, why? _____

_____

Major limitations of the study (2 or 3):

_____

_____

_____

Major strengths of the study (2 or 3):

_____

_____

_____

Are the results applicable or relevant to other settings, populations, or disciplines?

_____

_____

_____

USING RESEARCH RESULTS

Once you feel somewhat comfortable with the information in the article, ask yourself these questions:

Will information from the study help with the following?

Assessment:	Yes ❑	No ❑	Maybe ❑	Not applicable ❑
Procedure/protocol:	Yes ❑	No ❑	Maybe ❑	Not applicable ❑
Interventions:	Yes ❑	No ❑	Maybe ❑	Not applicable ❑
Interpersonal relationships:	Yes ❑	No ❑	Maybe ❑	Not applicable ❑
Quality improvement programs:	Yes ❑	No ❑	Maybe ❑	Not applicable ❑
Work life/environment:	Yes ❑	No ❑	Maybe ❑	Not applicable ❑
Education programs:	Yes ❑	No ❑	Maybe ❑	Not applicable ❑

Other:

_____

_____

Are the findings consistent with policies, procedures, and standards?

Require new policy:	Yes ❑	No ❑	Not sure ❑
Require new procedure:	Yes ❑	No ❑	Not sure ❑
Require new standard:	Yes ❑	No ❑	Not sure ❑
Can safety be maintained?	Yes ❑	No ❑	Not sure ❑

Do you think that the findings are acceptable to the following people?

Clients:	Yes ❏	No ❏	Not sure ❏
Administrators:	Yes ❏	No ❏	Not sure ❏
Colleagues:	Yes ❏	No ❏	Not sure ❏
Other professionals:	Yes ❏	No ❏	Not sure ❏

Are the following required for using the results?

Equipment:	Yes ❏	No ❏
Staff:	Yes ❏	No ❏
Time:	Yes ❏	No ❏
Money:	Yes ❏	No ❏
Knowledge/skills:	Yes ❏	No ❏
Attitude change:	Yes ❏	No ❏

Is the benefit worth the effort of obtaining the resources and changing practice?
Yes ❏   No ❏
Why or why not?

_____

_____